Methylene Blue Guide

Harnessing the Power of a Revolutionary Compound for Health and Wellness

Dr. Maxwell G. C. Philip

TABLE OF CONTENTS

Preface

Introduction to Methylene Blue

Methylene blue is one of the most remarkable substances in modern medicine and science. While it may sound like something pulled from the pages of a science fiction novel, this compound has been quietly changing lives for over a century. Originally synthesised in 1876 as a synthetic dye, methylene blue has evolved into a powerhouse in the world of biochemistry and medicine. Today, it is regarded not only as a diagnostic tool but also as a therapeutic agent capable of treating a wide range of conditions, from infections to neurodegenerative diseases.

At first glance, methylene blue may appear unassuming—just a blue dye used in laboratories, and more recently in diagnostic testing. However, its true power lies in its incredible impact on cellular health. Through its ability to improve mitochondrial function, methylene blue plays a critical role in addressing the root causes of many of the most chronic and debilitating diseases of our time.

In this book, I will take you on a journey through the science and history of methylene blue. You'll learn how this versatile compound works on a cellular level to improve your health in profound ways. From boosting energy levels and enhancing cognitive function to its potential in treating diseases such as cancer, Alzheimer's, and even viral infections, methylene blue offers a revolutionary approach to healing.

The Journey from Dye to Medicine

The story of methylene blue begins not in a laboratory, but in the textile industry. Originally, it was created as a synthetic dye in 1876 by the German chemist Heinrich Caro. Its blue pigment was quickly adopted in the textile industry for dyeing fabrics. However, scientists began to take notice of its unusual properties that went far beyond its use as a dye.

Methylene blue was found to have fascinating biological effects. In 1891, the first significant medical use of methylene blue was discovered when it was applied as a treatment for malaria. Researchers observed its ability to interfere with the malarial parasite, leading to a series of studies on its efficacy as an antimalarial drug. This marked the beginning of methylene blue's journey from a simple dye to a respected therapeutic tool.

As science advanced, researchers began to uncover methylene blue's broader potential. It was found to have the ability to improve cellular respiration, support mitochondrial function, and even act as an antioxidant. Its ability to enhance mitochondrial efficiency and energy production gave it an important role in the treatment of a variety of metabolic disorders. Over time, methylene blue was also identified as having neuroprotective properties, which led to its exploration as a potential treatment for neurodegenerative diseases like Alzheimer's.

In modern research, methylene blue has been the subject of numerous studies that have revealed its ability to improve cellular health, increase energy, alleviate pain, and combat mental health disorders. While it continues to be used in diagnostic imaging and medical treatments, its potential applications in a wide variety of therapeutic areas make it one of the most exciting substances in the world of medicine today.

Why This Book Matters: Harnessing the Power of Methylene Blue

As we move further into the 21st century, we are faced with an unprecedented rise in chronic diseases such as heart disease, diabetes, neurodegenerative diseases, and mental health disorders. While traditional medicine has made remarkable strides, many of these diseases remain difficult to treat and often progress despite our best efforts. The future of medicine, however, may lie in understanding the underlying metabolic processes that govern cellular health and discovering ways to optimise them.

This book is not just a technical exploration of methylene blue; it is a guide to unlocking its potential to revolutionise your health and well-being. By focusing on mitochondrial function and metabolic health, methylene blue represents a shift in how we approach disease and healing. As we explore the scientific basis of methylene blue's effects on the body, we will also explore its application in managing and even preventing conditions that have long been seen as incurable.

Through the chapters of this book, you will come to understand how methylene blue can be used to boost energy levels, enhance cognitive function, reduce inflammation, support cellular repair, and even provide a new line of defence against chronic diseases and infections.

One of the most compelling reasons to focus on methylene blue is its versatility. It is accessible, affordable, and, when used properly, safe. As an increasingly popular supplement, it has made its way into the hands of health-conscious individuals who are interested in optimising their well-being. However, the therapeutic benefits of methylene blue go beyond just a trendy supplement—it is a powerful tool that has the potential to transform our approach to health.

Why does this book matter? It matters because we are on the verge of a paradigm shift in how we understand health and disease. Methylene blue offers us a chance to look beyond symptomatic treatment and begin addressing the root causes of illness: mitochondrial dysfunction, metabolic imbalance, and cellular inefficiency. It offers a new way forward—a way that combines cutting-edge science with practical, actionable health strategies.

Whether you are suffering from a chronic illness, dealing with fatigue, or simply looking to improve your overall well-being, this book will provide you with the knowledge and tools to harness the power of methylene blue. You will gain insights into how this powerful compound works, how to use it safely, and how it can improve your quality of life. By the end of this book, you will have the information you need to make informed decisions about incorporating methylene blue into your health regimen.

Ultimately, this book is about empowerment—empowering you to take control of your health, explore alternative therapies, and harness the full potential of this extraordinary compound. Whether you're a health enthusiast, a practitioner, or someone looking for a new way to fight disease and improve vitality, the journey ahead will provide you with the tools to transform your health and your life.

Chapter 1: The Science of Methylene Blue

What is Methylene Blue?

Methylene blue (MB) is a chemical compound with the molecular formula **C16H18ClN3S**. It is a synthetic dye that appears as a deep blue colour in its crystalline form, hence the name "methylene blue." While it is often associated with its use in laboratories and as a diagnostic tool, it is far more than just a dye. Methylene blue is a remarkable substance with a wide range of biological effects that make it invaluable in medicine, biotechnology, and wellness.

Its chemical structure includes an aromatic ring system, a nitrogen atom in the central position, and a sulphur group, all of which contribute to its unique properties. The dye has been used for over a century in various applications, from staining tissue samples in laboratories to treating infections and neurological conditions.

In medicine, methylene blue is considered a redox agent—it has the ability to donate or accept electrons in biochemical reactions. This ability to participate in redox reactions is what gives methylene blue its therapeutic potential, especially in relation to mitochondrial function, which is central to energy production in cells. It has been found to have antioxidant, neuroprotective, and anti-inflammatory effects, making it an exciting tool in the treatment of diseases that involve cellular damage and mitochondrial dysfunction.

Although methylene blue was initially developed for use in the textile industry, where it was used as a dye for fabrics, its medicinal properties were soon discovered. Over the years, scientists have learned more about its effects on cellular energy production, mental clarity, and even its potential as a treatment for a variety of chronic diseases.

Historical Origins: From Textile Dye to Medical Miracle

The history of methylene blue dates back to 1876, when it was first synthesised by the German chemist Heinrich Caro. Initially, it was created as a synthetic dye used primarily in the textile industry for dyeing fabrics and as a biological stain for laboratory research. Its deep blue colour and ability to bind to tissues made it invaluable for scientific studies in histology and microbiology.

In the late 19th century, however, researchers began to explore the potential medicinal applications of methylene blue. One of the first major breakthroughs came in 1891 when researchers discovered that methylene blue could be used as a treatment for malaria. The compound was found to have the ability to interfere with the malarial parasite's ability to survive in the bloodstream, leading to a reduction in the symptoms of the disease. This early discovery of methylene blue's medical properties sparked a new wave of interest in its therapeutic potential.

During the 20th century, methylene blue continued to gain recognition for its uses in medical diagnostics, especially in its role as a vital stain for identifying bacterial infections and assessing tissue damage. However, it wasn't until the latter part of the century that researchers began to uncover its broader medical applications.

The discovery that methylene blue could have an effect on cellular respiration and mitochondrial function has been one of the most significant breakthroughs in understanding its potential therapeutic uses. As scientists began to learn more about the central role of mitochondria in health and disease, methylene blue emerged as a promising candidate for treating mitochondrial dysfunction, which is believed to be at the root of many chronic and degenerative diseases.

In modern medicine, methylene blue is used in a variety of therapeutic applications, including the treatment of methemoglobinemia (a condition in which the blood cannot effectively carry oxygen), as a diagnostic agent in imaging, and even as an adjunct in the treatment of neurological conditions like Alzheimer's and Parkinson's disease. It has gained attention in recent years for its potential to improve cellular energy, alleviate pain, and enhance cognitive function, making it a subject of intense research in the fields of ageing, metabolism, and mental health.

The Chemistry Behind Methylene Blue

Methylene blue is an organic compound that belongs to the family of heterocyclic aromatic compounds. Its structure consists of a thiazine ring, which contains nitrogen and sulphur atoms, and a benzene ring, which contributes to its stability and colour. This combination of rings forms a powerful redox-active system, making methylene blue an effective electron carrier in biochemical processes.

One of the key chemical properties of methylene blue is its ability to act as an electron donor or acceptor in biochemical reactions, particularly in cellular respiration. In this way, it plays a crucial role in supporting mitochondrial function by improving the efficiency of energy production.

Methylene blue's redox properties allow it to act as a reversible electron carrier in the electron transport chain (ETC), a series of reactions within mitochondria that are responsible for producing adenosine triphosphate (ATP), the cell's primary energy currency. In the electron transport chain, electrons are passed along a series of protein complexes, ultimately generating ATP. However, mitochondrial dysfunction can disrupt this process, leading to decreased energy production and the accumulation of harmful byproducts.

By intervening in this process, methylene blue can help restore the proper flow of electrons, enhancing mitochondrial efficiency and improving ATP production. This process is particularly beneficial in conditions where mitochondrial dysfunction is a primary contributor to disease, such as neurodegenerative disorders, metabolic diseases, and chronic fatigue syndrome.

Additionally, methylene blue is a potent antioxidant, which means it can neutralise free radicals—unstable molecules that can damage cells and contribute to ageing and disease. By reducing oxidative stress and promoting mitochondrial function, methylene blue helps to protect cells from damage and supports overall cellular health.

Methylene blue's chemical structure also allows it to cross the blood-brain barrier, making it a valuable tool in treating neurological disorders. Its ability to improve mitochondrial function in brain cells has been linked to enhanced cognitive function, better memory, and increased mental clarity. This has led to its exploration as a potential treatment for conditions like Alzheimer's disease, Parkinson's disease, and depression.

Understanding Mitochondrial Dysfunction and Metabolism

Mitochondria are the powerhouses of the cell, responsible for producing the energy necessary for nearly all cellular processes. They achieve this through a process known as oxidative phosphorylation, which occurs in the electron transport chain and generates ATP from the nutrients we consume. However, when mitochondria become damaged or dysfunctional, this energy production process is compromised, leading to a host of health issues.

Mitochondrial dysfunction is believed to be at the root of many chronic diseases, including neurodegenerative disorders like Alzheimer's and Parkinson's disease, metabolic conditions like diabetes, and even certain forms of cancer. As we age, mitochondrial function naturally declines, leading to reduced energy levels, increased oxidative stress, and a weakened ability to repair cellular damage. This decline in mitochondrial health is also associated with a number of age-related conditions, including cognitive decline, muscle weakness, and chronic fatigue.

One of the most groundbreaking aspects of methylene blue is its ability to restore mitochondrial function. By enhancing the efficiency of the electron transport chain, methylene blue helps mitochondria produce more energy, thus improving overall cellular function. This has profound implications for treating diseases that stem from mitochondrial dysfunction. For instance, in neurodegenerative diseases like Alzheimer's, where brain cells suffer from impaired energy production, methylene blue's ability to improve mitochondrial activity can help protect neurons, enhance cognitive function, and slow disease progression.

Additionally, methylene blue's antioxidant properties further support cellular health by reducing oxidative stress, which can damage mitochondria and other cell structures. By neutralising harmful free radicals, methylene blue protects cells from the kind of damage that accelerates ageing and contributes to chronic disease.

In terms of metabolism, mitochondrial health is essential for maintaining balanced energy levels throughout the day. When mitochondria function optimally, they help regulate the body's metabolism, supporting efficient fat burning, glucose utilisation, and energy expenditure. Methylene blue's ability to enhance mitochondrial function can therefore improve metabolism, aid in weight management, and increase energy levels.

Chapter 2: Mitochondria – The Powerhouses of Our Cells

The Role of Mitochondria in Health and Disease

Mitochondria are often referred to as the "powerhouses" of our cells because they are responsible for producing the majority of the energy our bodies require. These tiny, membrane-bound organelles are found in almost every cell of the body, with the exception of red blood cells, and are essential for normal cellular function and survival. Mitochondria convert the nutrients we consume, primarily glucose and fats, into adenosine triphosphate (ATP), which is the energy currency of the cell. ATP fuels a wide variety of cellular processes, including muscle contractions, nerve impulses, protein synthesis, and other essential functions that sustain life.

Mitochondria are complex structures with their own DNA, which is distinct from the DNA in the nucleus of the cell. This mitochondrial DNA (mtDNA) is inherited maternally and encodes for some of the proteins that are involved in mitochondrial function. Unlike other organelles, mitochondria have the ability to divide and replicate themselves, allowing them to respond to the changing energy needs of the body.

The mitochondria's primary role is in cellular respiration—a process by which cells generate ATP through a series of biochemical reactions. These reactions occur in the mitochondria and are responsible for producing energy from the food we eat. The mitochondria play a central role in many biological processes, including:

1. **Energy production:** ATP is the key energy molecule that powers cellular activities.

2. **Regulation of cell death (apoptosis):** Mitochondria are involved in triggering the programmed cell death process when cells are damaged beyond repair. This is essential for maintaining cellular health and preventing the proliferation of damaged cells.

3. **Calcium regulation:** Mitochondria help regulate calcium levels within the cell, which is important for processes such as muscle contraction, neurotransmission, and the regulation of enzyme activity.

4. **Heat production (thermogenesis):** In certain tissues like brown adipose tissue, mitochondria are involved in heat production, which helps regulate body temperature.

The efficiency of mitochondrial function is paramount for overall health. When mitochondria perform their functions optimally, the body has sufficient energy for all its activities, from basic cellular processes to complex physical movements. Conversely, when mitochondrial function is compromised, it can lead to a variety of health problems.

Mitochondrial Dysfunction: The Root of Many Chronic Conditions

Mitochondrial dysfunction occurs when the mitochondria's ability to produce energy is impaired, leading to cellular inefficiency, increased oxidative stress, and a breakdown in the normal functioning of the cells. Mitochondrial dysfunction is believed to be at the root of many chronic diseases, including neurological disorders, metabolic diseases, and even cancer.

As we age, the number and functionality of mitochondria naturally decline. This process is linked to the ageing of cells and tissues, contributing to the development of age-related diseases and conditions. However, mitochondrial dysfunction can also occur prematurely due to genetic mutations, lifestyle factors (such as poor diet and lack of exercise), toxins, and chronic stress.

Some of the chronic conditions associated with mitochondrial dysfunction include:

1. **Neurodegenerative Diseases:** Mitochondrial dysfunction has been implicated in various neurodegenerative disorders, such as Alzheimer's disease, Parkinson's disease, Huntington's disease, and Amyotrophic Lateral Sclerosis (ALS). In these conditions, the brain's cells, which rely heavily on mitochondria for energy, suffer from a lack of energy, causing cell death, cognitive decline, and motor dysfunction.

2. **Metabolic Diseases:** Mitochondrial dysfunction is a key player in metabolic disorders such as obesity, diabetes, and insulin resistance. Since mitochondria are

responsible for converting food into energy, when they are not functioning properly, it can lead to poor energy utilisation, weight gain, and increased risk of developing type 2 diabetes.

3. **Cardiovascular Disease:** Mitochondria play a crucial role in heart function, as heart muscle cells require large amounts of energy to maintain their pumping action. Mitochondrial dysfunction in heart cells can lead to conditions such as heart failure and ischemic heart disease.

4. **Cancer:** Abnormal mitochondrial function is also linked to the development and progression of cancer. Cancer cells often exhibit altered mitochondrial metabolism, a phenomenon known as the Warburg effect, where cancer cells prefer to generate energy through anaerobic glycolysis rather than oxidative phosphorylation, even when oxygen is available. This shift in metabolism contributes to uncontrolled cell growth, a hallmark of cancer.

5. **Chronic Fatigue Syndrome and Fibromyalgia:** These conditions are thought to be related to impaired mitochondrial function. The reduced ability to produce ATP can result in chronic feelings of fatigue, muscle weakness, and pain.

6. **Ageing:** As mitochondrial function declines with age, the ability to produce ATP diminishes, leading to reduced energy, cognitive decline, and the gradual breakdown of tissues and organs. This process contributes to the development of many age-related conditions.

Mitochondrial dysfunction leads to a vicious cycle of decreased energy production, increased oxidative stress, and cellular damage. Oxidative stress refers to an imbalance between the production of free radicals (reactive oxygen species, or ROS) and the body's ability to neutralise them with antioxidants. When mitochondria are damaged, they generate excess ROS, which can further damage mitochondrial components and other cellular structures. This cycle of damage and dysfunction is a contributing factor to the development of many chronic and degenerative diseases.

How Methylene Blue Interacts with Mitochondria

Methylene blue is one of the few compounds that have been found to directly interact with mitochondria to improve their function. It has the remarkable ability to enhance mitochondrial efficiency, boost ATP production, and reduce oxidative stress—all of which contribute to improved cellular health.

1. **Mitochondrial Electron Transport Chain (ETC) Enhancement:** Methylene blue acts as a **redox mediator**, meaning it can transfer electrons between molecules, facilitating the flow of electrons through the mitochondrial electron transport chain (ETC). The ETC is responsible for generating ATP through oxidative phosphorylation. By improving the

efficiency of this process, methylene blue increases ATP production, giving cells the energy they need to function properly. This is especially beneficial for tissues and organs that have high energy demands, such as the brain, heart, and muscles.

2. **Antioxidant Properties:** Methylene blue also has potent **antioxidant effects**, helping to neutralise the excess reactive oxygen species (ROS) that are produced during cellular respiration. ROS can damage mitochondrial components and other cellular structures, leading to further dysfunction. By reducing oxidative stress, methylene blue protects mitochondria and other cells from damage, which can slow down the ageing process and help prevent chronic diseases.

3. **Neuroprotective Effects:** Since the brain requires an enormous amount of energy to function, methylene blue's ability to enhance mitochondrial function has neuroprotective benefits. It helps to

support cognitive function, improve memory, and potentially prevent neurodegenerative diseases like Alzheimer's and Parkinson's disease. The improvement in mitochondrial function helps the brain cells generate more ATP, which is crucial for mental clarity and cognitive health.

4. **Increased Cellular Respiration:** By enhancing mitochondrial respiration, methylene blue increases the overall metabolic activity of cells. This leads to improved energy production, which benefits every tissue and organ in the body, promoting overall health and vitality. For people with conditions like chronic fatigue syndrome or fibromyalgia, methylene blue's effect on mitochondrial function can help alleviate symptoms of fatigue and muscle weakness.

5. **Mitochondrial Biogenesis:** Research has shown that methylene blue can stimulate the process of **mitochondrial biogenesis**, which is the creation of new mitochondria

within cells. This is an important mechanism for maintaining healthy mitochondrial populations, especially when existing mitochondria are damaged or inefficient. Methylene blue may help to rejuvenate ageing tissues and promote the growth of new, functional mitochondria.

The Science of Cellular Energy and ATP Production

At the heart of mitochondrial function is the production of **ATP**, the molecule that powers nearly every cellular process. ATP is produced through two primary pathways in the mitochondria: **glycolysis** and **oxidative phosphorylation**.

- **Glycolysis**: This occurs in the cytoplasm and is the first step in the breakdown of glucose to produce ATP. While glycolysis is less efficient than oxidative phosphorylation, it is an essential process for energy production, particularly in conditions where oxygen supply is limited.

- **Oxidative Phosphorylation (OxPhos):** This occurs in the mitochondria and involves a complex series of reactions known as the electron transport chain. Electrons from nutrients (like glucose and fatty acids) are transferred through protein complexes in the mitochondrial inner membrane, ultimately creating a proton gradient that drives the production of ATP. This process is highly efficient and produces the bulk of the ATP needed by cells for normal functioning.

The mitochondria's ability to produce ATP depends on the efficiency of the electron transport chain and the availability of nutrients, such as oxygen and glucose. When mitochondrial function is impaired, ATP production is reduced, leading to a variety of symptoms associated with fatigue, cognitive decline, muscle weakness, and other health issues. Methylene blue acts as a key player in enhancing this process, ensuring that the mitochondria can continue to generate ATP efficiently and restore energy levels to the cells.

Chapter 3: Methylene Blue and Its Therapeutic Benefits

Methylene blue, a compound originally developed as a dye, has gained widespread attention for its remarkable therapeutic effects. Over time, it has been discovered that methylene blue has the potential to revolutionise health care by addressing a wide range of health conditions. From boosting cellular energy to enhancing mental clarity, accelerating recovery from injuries, improving mood, and even optimising sexual health, methylene blue is emerging as a powerful ally in modern medicine.

Boosting Cellular Energy: How Methylene Blue Revitalizes the Body

One of the primary mechanisms through which methylene blue exerts its therapeutic effects is by boosting cellular energy. The mitochondria, often referred to as the "powerhouses" of our cells, are responsible for producing energy in the form of adenosine triphosphate (ATP). However, mitochondrial function can decline due to factors such as ageing, stress, poor nutrition, and disease, leading to a decrease in ATP production. This lack of energy manifests as fatigue, cognitive impairment, and poor physical performance.

Methylene blue plays a crucial role in revitalising the body by enhancing mitochondrial function and increasing ATP production. The compound acts as a **redox mediator**, facilitating the flow of electrons through the mitochondrial electron transport chain (ETC). This action improves the efficiency of oxidative phosphorylation, the process by which mitochondria generate ATP. As a result, methylene blue helps to restore energy production in cells, which can alleviate fatigue and improve overall vitality.

Additionally, methylene blue's antioxidant properties reduce oxidative stress, which occurs when the body is overwhelmed by free radicals and reactive oxygen species (ROS). These harmful molecules can damage cellular structures, impair mitochondrial function, and contribute to the development of chronic diseases. By neutralising free radicals, methylene blue protects mitochondria and other cells from damage, further supporting energy production and overall health.

The ability of methylene blue to boost cellular energy has far-reaching effects on the body. Enhanced ATP production improves physical performance, mental clarity, and stamina, making it particularly beneficial for individuals experiencing fatigue-related conditions, such as chronic fatigue syndrome, fibromyalgia, or post-viral fatigue.

Brain Function and Mental Clarity: Enhancing Cognitive Performance

Methylene blue's effects on brain function are some of its most celebrated benefits. The brain is one of the most energy-demanding organs in the body, requiring a constant supply of ATP to maintain cognitive function. Mitochondria in brain cells, particularly in neurons, are responsible for generating the energy needed for thinking, memory, concentration, and learning. When mitochondrial function is compromised, cognitive performance can suffer, leading to issues like memory loss, lack of focus, and mental fog.

Methylene blue has been shown to improve brain function by enhancing mitochondrial efficiency in neurons, which directly translates to better cognitive performance. By increasing ATP production in the brain, methylene blue helps support mental clarity, memory, and learning ability. This is particularly valuable for individuals experiencing age-related cognitive decline or neurodegenerative diseases like Alzheimer's and Parkinson's disease.

Research has demonstrated that methylene blue's neuroprotective effects may also extend to **brain cell protection**. It has been shown to reduce oxidative stress and promote the health of neurons by inhibiting the formation of harmful proteins that can lead to neurodegeneration. This makes methylene blue a potential therapeutic agent in the prevention and management of cognitive disorders.

Additionally, methylene blue has been found to enhance **neuroplasticity**, the brain's ability to reorganise and form new neural connections. This is particularly beneficial for individuals recovering from brain injuries, strokes, or traumatic events that affect cognitive function. By promoting neuroplasticity, methylene blue helps the brain adapt and heal, potentially improving outcomes for patients with brain trauma or chronic neurodegenerative conditions.

In essence, methylene blue offers a multifaceted approach to improving cognitive function. It boosts energy production in brain cells, protects neurons from damage, and promotes the regeneration of new neural pathways, all of which contribute to enhanced memory, focus, and mental clarity.

Pain Relief and Injury Healing: Accelerating Recovery

Methylene blue's ability to accelerate the body's healing processes makes it an effective therapeutic agent for pain relief and injury recovery. One of the ways it achieves this is by improving cellular energy production. In the case of injury or trauma, the body requires a significant amount of energy to repair tissues, regenerate cells, and combat inflammation. Mitochondrial dysfunction can hinder the body's ability to generate the ATP needed for these processes, leading to delayed recovery and prolonged pain.

By enhancing mitochondrial function and increasing ATP production, methylene blue helps to speed up recovery from injury. It supports the repair of damaged tissues and promotes the regeneration of healthy cells, leading to faster healing times. This is particularly valuable for individuals recovering from **sports injuries, surgery, or trauma**, as well as those with chronic pain conditions like osteoarthritis or fibromyalgia.

Moreover, methylene blue's **anti-inflammatory** properties further contribute to pain relief. Inflammation is a natural response to injury, but chronic inflammation can lead to prolonged pain and tissue damage. Methylene blue has been shown to reduce inflammation, which can help alleviate pain and promote healing. Its antioxidant properties also play a role in reducing oxidative stress and cellular damage, which can further improve recovery outcomes.

Methylene blue's potential to accelerate injury healing and alleviate pain is supported by research in both animal and human studies. For example, it has been shown to improve **muscle recovery** and reduce muscle fatigue following intense physical exertion. This makes it particularly useful for athletes or individuals undergoing physical rehabilitation.

Elevating Mood: Combatting Depression and Anxiety

Mental health conditions, such as depression and anxiety, are prevalent in today's society and can have a profound impact on an individual's quality of life. The conventional treatments for these conditions often involve medication that targets neurotransmitter imbalances in the brain, but these treatments can have side effects and may not work for everyone. Methylene blue offers a novel approach to improving mood and emotional well-being.

Methylene blue has been found to have **antidepressant** and **anxiolytic**

(anxiety-reducing) effects through several mechanisms. One of the primary ways it achieves this is by enhancing mitochondrial function in brain cells. As discussed earlier, mitochondria are responsible for producing the energy required for cellular processes, including neurotransmitter production and regulation. When mitochondrial function is impaired, it can lead to dysregulation of neurotransmitters, contributing to mood disorders such as depression and anxiety.

By improving mitochondrial efficiency and increasing ATP production in the brain, methylene blue helps to restore balance to neurotransmitter systems, which may alleviate symptoms of depression and anxiety. Additionally, methylene blue's antioxidant properties reduce oxidative stress in the brain, which has been linked to the development of mood disorders. Oxidative stress can damage neurons and disrupt the signalling pathways that regulate mood, making it more difficult for the brain to maintain emotional stability.

Methylene blue has also been shown to **increase serotonin** levels in the brain, a neurotransmitter that plays a key role in regulating mood, sleep, and appetite. Low levels of serotonin are often associated with depression, so increasing serotonin availability may improve mood and alleviate symptoms of depression.

For individuals struggling with depression and anxiety, methylene blue offers a promising alternative or complement to traditional therapies. Its ability to enhance mitochondrial function, reduce oxidative stress, and regulate neurotransmitter activity makes it a powerful tool for supporting emotional well-being.

Sexual Health: Enhancing Libido, Fertility, and Performance

Methylene blue has also shown potential benefits in the realm of sexual health. Sexual function is closely tied to mitochondrial health, as the energy produced by mitochondria is essential for the proper functioning of reproductive organs and sexual tissues.

Mitochondrial dysfunction can impair circulation, hormone production, and nerve function, leading to issues such as low libido, erectile dysfunction, and fertility problems.

By boosting ATP production in the mitochondria, methylene blue helps to support sexual health in several key ways:

1. **Improved Blood Flow and Circulation:** Mitochondrial energy is required for the proper functioning of blood vessels, including those that supply the genital area. By enhancing mitochondrial function, methylene blue improves circulation, which can lead to better sexual performance and increased libido.

2. **Enhanced Fertility:** Mitochondria are involved in the production of hormones such as testosterone and oestrogen, which are critical for sexual function and fertility. By improving mitochondrial efficiency, methylene blue supports hormone production and may help address issues related to infertility.

3. **Erectile Function and Libido:** In men, mitochondrial dysfunction in penile tissue can contribute to erectile dysfunction (ED). Methylene blue's ability to enhance mitochondrial function and improve blood flow may help alleviate symptoms of ED, improve erectile function, and increase libido.

4. **Increased Stamina and Sexual Performance:** By boosting overall energy levels and reducing fatigue, methylene blue can enhance sexual stamina and performance, leading to a more satisfying sexual experience.

In women, methylene blue's benefits for sexual health extend to increased vaginal lubrication, improved sexual response, and enhanced libido, all of which contribute to a healthier and more fulfilling sexual life.

Chapter 4: Methylene Blue and Its Role in Disease Prevention

Methylene blue, a compound once used primarily as a dye in the textile industry, has evolved into a therapeutic agent with broad implications for disease prevention and treatment. As research into its mechanisms of action continues to unfold, the compound has gained recognition for its ability to target the root causes of many chronic and acute health conditions. From viral infections and cancer to neurodegenerative diseases and cardiovascular health, methylene blue demonstrates significant potential in preventing and managing a variety of diseases.

The Power of Methylene Blue Against Viruses (COVID, AIDS, and More)

In recent years, methylene blue has attracted considerable attention for its antiviral properties, particularly in the context of emerging viruses such as **COVID-19** and **HIV/AIDS**. Methylene blue's ability to fight viruses lies in its multifaceted approach to cellular and viral biology. As a **photosensitizer**, methylene blue can generate reactive oxygen species (ROS) when exposed to light, which can damage the viral structure and inhibit viral replication. This ability has been explored in several studies, with methylene blue demonstrating the potential to **inactivate viruses** in vitro and prevent their spread.

In the case of **COVID-19**, researchers have begun investigating the potential of methylene blue as a **treatment option**. The virus responsible for COVID-19, SARS-CoV-2, primarily targets the respiratory system but also has systemic effects that may involve the cardiovascular and neurological systems. Methylene blue has shown promise in laboratory studies by **disrupting the viral envelope** and hindering the virus's ability to infect host cells. Moreover, its **antioxidant and anti-inflammatory properties** could mitigate some of the systemic damage caused by COVID-19, particularly in individuals experiencing long-term symptoms such as fatigue, brain fog, and lung damage.

Methylene blue's potential antiviral benefits are not limited to COVID-19. The compound has also demonstrated effectiveness against **HIV**, the virus responsible for **AIDS**. HIV attacks the immune system, leading to a weakened defence against other infections and diseases. Methylene blue has been shown to **inhibit HIV replication,** thereby reducing the viral load in individuals infected with the virus. By **enhancing mitochondrial function**, methylene blue may also help bolster the immune response, making the body better equipped to fight off infections, including those caused by HIV.

Furthermore, methylene blue's **anti-inflammatory** effects could help reduce the chronic inflammation that is often associated with viral infections. Chronic inflammation contributes to a variety of health problems, including **autoimmune disorders**, **cardiovascular disease**, and **neurodegeneration**. By mitigating inflammation, methylene blue may play a crucial role in preventing viral-related complications and improving overall health.

Methylene Blue in Cancer Treatment: Fighting Cells at the Source

Cancer remains one of the most devastating diseases worldwide, characterised by uncontrolled cell growth and the spread of malignant cells to other parts of the body. Current cancer treatments, such as chemotherapy and radiation, aim to kill cancerous cells but can also damage healthy cells, leading to severe side effects. Methylene blue, however, offers a novel approach to cancer treatment, potentially providing a safer and more effective alternative or adjunct therapy.

Methylene blue works in cancer treatment by targeting the **metabolic dysfunction** that is often present in cancer cells. Cancer cells, unlike normal cells, tend to rely on **anaerobic metabolism** (metabolism without oxygen) for energy production, even in the presence of oxygen. This phenomenon, known as the **Warburg effect**, makes cancer cells more dependent on glycolysis (the breakdown of glucose) and less efficient at using oxygen to produce ATP. Methylene blue's ability to enhance mitochondrial function and promote **aerobic metabolism** can help restore the balance of energy production in cells, potentially starving cancer cells of the energy they need to survive and proliferate.

Moreover, methylene blue has been shown to **induce apoptosis** (programmed cell death) in cancer cells, which is a critical mechanism for eliminating abnormal cells. By triggering the intrinsic apoptotic pathway, methylene blue can encourage the self-destruction of cancer cells without harming surrounding healthy tissues. This is a highly beneficial property, as it could help minimise the side effects typically associated with chemotherapy and radiation therapy.

In addition to its effects on cancer cell metabolism, methylene blue's **anti-inflammatory** and **antioxidant** properties could help to counteract the chronic inflammation and oxidative stress often seen in cancer. Chronic inflammation can promote tumour growth, metastasis, and resistance to treatment, so by reducing this inflammation, methylene blue may assist in limiting cancer progression and improving the effectiveness of other therapies.

While research into methylene blue's role in cancer treatment is still in its early stages, preliminary studies suggest that it could be a valuable tool in the fight against cancer, particularly when used in conjunction with other treatment modalities.

Alzheimer's and Neurodegeneration: Protecting the Brain

Alzheimer's disease, Parkinson's disease, and other neurodegenerative conditions are on the rise as the global population ages. These diseases are characterised by the progressive degeneration of neurons in the brain, leading to cognitive decline, memory loss, and motor dysfunction. Although there is no cure for these diseases, emerging therapies like methylene blue are showing promise in **protecting the brain** and slowing the progression of neurodegeneration.

Methylene blue's neuroprotective properties stem from its ability to **improve mitochondrial function** in brain cells. Mitochondria are critical for neuronal health, as they supply the energy needed for neurotransmission and cell maintenance. In neurodegenerative diseases, mitochondrial dysfunction is a common feature, contributing to neuronal death and cognitive decline. By enhancing mitochondrial activity, methylene blue supports brain cell survival and function, potentially delaying or halting the progression of Alzheimer's, Parkinson's, and other neurodegenerative diseases.

Moreover, methylene blue has been shown to **reduce the accumulation of toxic proteins** such as beta-amyloid, which is commonly associated with Alzheimer's disease. The buildup of beta-amyloid plaques in the brain disrupts neuronal communication and leads to cognitive decline. Methylene blue may help prevent the formation of these plaques, reducing the neurotoxic effects they have on the brain.

Methylene blue also possesses **antioxidant properties** that can help protect neurons from oxidative stress, a key factor in the development of Alzheimer's and other neurodegenerative diseases. By neutralising free radicals and preventing oxidative damage, methylene blue helps maintain brain health and function.

In addition to its effects on mitochondrial function and oxidative stress, methylene blue has shown promise in improving **cognitive performance** in individuals with Alzheimer's disease. Clinical studies have suggested that methylene blue can enhance memory, focus, and overall cognitive abilities, potentially providing a much-needed therapeutic option for individuals with neurodegenerative conditions.

Autism Spectrum Disorder: Possible Benefits and Controversies

Autism Spectrum Disorder (ASD) is a complex neurodevelopmental condition that affects an individual's social interactions, communication skills, and behaviour. The causes of autism are not yet fully understood, but it is believed to involve a combination of genetic, environmental, and neurological factors. Some researchers have explored the potential benefits of methylene blue for individuals with ASD, particularly in relation to mitochondrial dysfunction and brain health.

Mitochondrial dysfunction has been observed in individuals with autism, and enhancing mitochondrial function may have a positive effect on **neurological development** and **behavioural function**. Methylene blue's ability to improve mitochondrial efficiency in brain cells could help restore normal neurological function, potentially improving communication, social interactions, and cognitive abilities in individuals with autism.

Additionally, methylene blue's **anti-inflammatory** and **neuroprotective** effects may play a role in reducing the neurological symptoms of autism. Some studies have shown that inflammation in the brain is linked to the severity of autism symptoms, and by reducing this inflammation, methylene blue could help alleviate certain behavioural challenges associated with the condition.

However, the use of methylene blue for autism is still a topic of **controversy** and ongoing research. While some studies suggest potential benefits, others caution that the compound may have side effects or interactions with medications commonly used to treat autism. It is essential that any potential use of methylene blue for autism be carefully considered and discussed with a healthcare professional.

Cardiovascular Health: Supporting the Heart and Circulation

Methylene blue's therapeutic effects extend to cardiovascular health, where it plays a role in **enhancing circulation**, **improving blood flow**, and **supporting heart function**. The heart and blood vessels are highly dependent on mitochondrial energy to maintain their function. Mitochondrial dysfunction in cardiovascular cells can lead to a variety of heart-related problems, including **heart failure**, **arterial plaque buildup**, and **hypertension**.

Methylene blue can help restore normal mitochondrial function in heart cells, improving the heart's ability to pump blood efficiently and maintain proper circulation. By enhancing mitochondrial energy production, methylene blue supports **cardiovascular endurance**, which is particularly beneficial for individuals with **heart disease** or **circulatory problems**.

Moreover, methylene blue has been shown to possess **vasodilatory** properties, meaning that it can help relax and widen blood vessels, thereby improving blood flow and lowering blood pressure. This effect makes methylene blue a potential adjunct therapy for individuals with **hypertension** or poor circulation.

Additionally, methylene blue's **antioxidant** and **anti-inflammatory** properties contribute to cardiovascular health by reducing oxidative stress and inflammation in blood vessels and the heart. Chronic inflammation in the cardiovascular system is a major contributor to atherosclerosis (plaque buildup in the arteries), which can lead to heart attacks and strokes. By reducing inflammation, methylene blue may help prevent or manage cardiovascular diseases.

Chapter 5: How to Safely Use Methylene Blue

Methylene blue has gained significant attention for its therapeutic potential in treating a variety of health conditions, from enhancing cognitive function to combating infections and even supporting cardiovascular health. However, like any powerful compound, its benefits must be balanced with safety considerations. To maximise the therapeutic effects of methylene blue while minimising potential risks, it is essential to understand the appropriate dosages, forms, side effects, and precautions associated with its use.

Recommended Dosage and Administration Guidelines

The appropriate dosage of methylene blue depends on various factors, including the specific health condition being treated, the form of methylene blue being used, and individual factors such as age, weight, and overall health. The following guidelines provide a general framework for **safe use** of methylene blue, but it is crucial to consult with a healthcare provider before beginning any treatment regimen.

1. **Standard Dosing for Cognitive Enhancement**:
   - **Low doses (0.5–4 mg/kg)**: For cognitive and brain health benefits, methylene blue is typically used in lower doses. In clinical trials, **0.5–4 mg per kilogram** of body weight has been found to improve mitochondrial function, enhance memory, and protect against neurodegenerative diseases without significant adverse effects.

- For example, a person weighing 70 kg (around 154 lbs) would generally take **35–280 mg** of methylene blue per day. However, the lower end of the dose range (e.g., 35 mg per day) is recommended to start with to assess individual tolerance.

2. **Dosing for Antiviral and Anti-Cancer Effects**:
   - **Higher doses (4–8 mg/kg)**: For more severe conditions, such as viral infections or cancer treatment, higher doses may be appropriate. Doses between **4–8 mg/kg** per day are commonly used in clinical studies investigating methylene blue's effects on these diseases.
   - For example, a 70 kg individual might take **280–560 mg** per day, though these doses are typically administered under medical supervision to monitor safety and efficacy.

3. **Acute Treatment and Injections**:
   - In emergency settings, such as **methemoglobinemia (a condition in which the blood cannot carry oxygen efficiently)**, methylene blue may be administered intravenously at a **dose of 1–2 mg/kg**. This administration should only occur under medical supervision, typically in a hospital or clinic, as intravenous administration carries specific risks that need to be carefully monitored.

It is crucial to **start with lower doses** and gradually increase as needed, especially for individuals using methylene blue for cognitive enhancement or chronic conditions. Always adjust the dose based on how your body responds and consult with a healthcare provider if any side effects occur.

Forms of Methylene Blue: Supplements, Injections, and More

Methylene blue is available in several forms, each with its own specific use cases, dosages, and administration methods. Understanding these different forms is crucial for selecting the best option for your needs.

1. **Oral Supplements (Tablets and Powders)**:
   - **Methylene Blue Tablets**: The most common and accessible form of methylene blue for general use is in **tablet form**. These are available in various strengths, typically ranging from **5 mg to 100 mg per tablet**. Oral tablets are convenient for those seeking to use methylene blue for cognitive enhancement, mood elevation, or other therapeutic purposes.
   - **Methylene Blue Powders**: For more customised dosages, **methylene blue powder** is available and can be dissolved in water or another beverage. This

allows for more flexibility in dosing but requires accurate measurement for safety.

2. **Methylene Blue Injections**:
   o In clinical settings, **methylene blue is often administered intravenously (IV),** especially in emergency situations like treating **methemoglobinemia** or specific cases of **infection**. This method requires careful medical supervision, as the IV form delivers a **higher concentration of methylene blue directly into the bloodstream**, leading to quicker therapeutic effects.
   o Injection forms are usually prescribed by healthcare professionals for acute treatments and should only be administered under **medical supervision**.

3. **Topical Use (Less Common)**:
   o Methylene blue is sometimes used in topical applications, particularly

in **wound care** or as a **disinfectant**. For instance, it has been used to treat **skin infections**, **ulcers**, and **burns** due to its antiseptic properties. However, this form of methylene blue is typically used in specific clinical contexts and is not recommended for general health purposes without professional oversight.

4. **Nasal Sprays (Emerging Form)**:
    ○ An emerging form of methylene blue for **neuroprotection** and **cognitive function** enhancement is a **nasal spray**. This method is gaining attention for its potential to deliver the compound **directly to the brain** through the olfactory system, bypassing the digestive system and offering faster absorption. Research into the effectiveness and safety of this form is still in its early stages, but it

holds promise for future therapeutic use.

Potential Side Effects and How to Mitigate Risks

While methylene blue has shown a remarkable safety profile in many studies, like any therapeutic agent, it does carry the risk of side effects, particularly when used inappropriately or at high doses. Awareness of these potential side effects and strategies for **mitigating risks** can help ensure a safer experience with methylene blue.

1. **Common Side Effects**:
   - **Urine Discoloration**: One of the most notable side effects of methylene blue is its ability to turn urine a **blue or green colour**. This is harmless and simply the result of the body excreting the compound. It does not require medical intervention and typically resolves once methylene blue is metabolised.

- **Digestive Upset**: Some individuals may experience **nausea**, **vomiting**, or **stomach discomfort** when taking methylene blue orally. To mitigate this, it is recommended to take methylene blue with food or to start with a smaller dose to allow the body to adjust.
- **Headaches and Dizziness**: In some cases, methylene blue may cause **headaches** or **dizziness**, especially if taken at high doses. Reducing the dose or discontinuing use can often alleviate these symptoms.

2. **Serious Side Effects**:
   - **Serotonin Syndrome**: When taken with medications that increase serotonin levels (e.g., **selective serotonin reuptake inhibitors (SSRIs)** or **monoamine oxidase inhibitors (MAOIs))**, methylene blue can interact to cause **serotonin syndrome**, a potentially life-threatening condition

characterised by agitation,
confusion, rapid heart rate, high
blood pressure, and fever. To
minimise this risk, **avoid
combining methylene blue** with
serotonergic medications unless
under strict medical supervision.

- **Methemoglobinemia**:
  Paradoxically, although methylene
  blue is used to **treat
  methemoglobinemia**, high doses of
  methylene blue in some individuals
  may actually cause it. Symptoms
  include cyanosis (a bluish tint to the
  skin) and shortness of breath. This
  is a rare side effect and is typically
  associated with higher doses.
  Monitoring oxygen levels and
  seeking medical advice can help
  mitigate this risk.

3. **How to Mitigate Risks**:
   - **Start with Low Doses**: Always
     begin with the **lowest possible dose**
     of methylene blue, especially if you

are new to the compound. Gradually increase the dose as needed while observing how your body responds.

○ **Monitor Drug Interactions**: Be aware of any medications you are taking and consult with your healthcare provider to ensure that methylene blue will not interact negatively with them, particularly those that influence serotonin levels or blood pressure.

○ **Hydration**: Ensure that you stay well-hydrated while using methylene blue, especially if you are taking higher doses. This will help your body process and eliminate the compound more effectively.

Safety Precautions and Medical Oversight

Due to the potency of methylene blue, it is highly recommended to use it **under medical supervision**, especially for high doses or for individuals with underlying health conditions. Here are some important safety precautions to consider:

- **Consult a Healthcare Provider**: Before beginning any form of methylene blue therapy, it is crucial to consult with a healthcare provider, particularly if you have any pre-existing conditions, are pregnant or breastfeeding, or are taking medications for other conditions.
- **Regular Monitoring**: If using methylene blue for chronic conditions or at higher doses, regular monitoring of vital signs, including blood pressure, heart rate, and oxygen levels, is recommended. This is especially important if using methylene blue in conjunction with other medications.
- **Avoid Self-Medicating for Serious Conditions**: While methylene blue has therapeutic potential, it should not be used as a sole treatment for serious medical conditions (such as cancer or viral

infections) without the guidance of a healthcare provider. It is best used as a complementary treatment, not a replacement for standard medical care.

Best Practices for Long-Term Use

If you plan to use methylene blue over an extended period, follow these best practices to ensure safe and effective use:

1. **Cycle Use**: If using methylene blue for cognitive enhancement or other long-term benefits, it is recommended to **cycle** its use. For instance, use it for 4-6 weeks, followed by a 1-2 week break. This helps to prevent any potential tolerance buildup and ensures continued effectiveness.

2. **Dosage Adjustments**: Over time, the body may adjust to methylene blue, and the initial dose may become less effective. Periodically reassess the dosage with your healthcare provider to ensure optimal benefits.

3. **Healthy Lifestyle**: Support the effects of methylene blue with a healthy diet, regular exercise, and proper sleep hygiene. This will help maximise its therapeutic effects and contribute to overall well-being.

Chapter 6: Methylene Blue in Alternative Medicine

Methylene blue is often viewed as a chemical compound with significant medical potential, but its integration into **alternative and holistic medicine** presents a fascinating paradigm shift. Many alternative health practitioners and individuals seeking complementary therapies are exploring how methylene blue can be used alongside or instead of conventional treatments.

Integrating Methylene Blue into Holistic Health Practices

Holistic health practices focus on treating the body, mind, and spirit as an interconnected whole. They prioritise **natural, non-invasive treatments** to encourage self-healing, and methylene blue is increasingly seen as a promising addition to these practices. From its ability to enhance **mitochondrial function** and **boost energy levels** to its potential to combat **cognitive decline**, methylene blue aligns with several principles of holistic healing.

1. **Mitochondrial Support and Energy Revitalization**: One of the primary uses of methylene blue in holistic practices is its role in **cellular energy production**. In alternative medicine, mitochondrial health is often emphasised as a cornerstone for overall vitality. Methylene blue is known to promote the efficient functioning of **mitochondria**, the powerhouses of our cells, and improve **ATP production**, which leads to more energy. This makes it a great adjunct for those seeking natural methods to boost **energy**, combat **fatigue**,

or **revitalise** their bodies. It can be incorporated into detox regimens or used in conjunction with other supplements designed to support cellular health.

2. **Cognitive Health and Mental Clarity**: Holistic practitioners often emphasise the use of natural nootropics, or cognitive enhancers, to promote mental clarity and brain health. Methylene blue fits well within this approach due to its well-documented effects on **brain function**, from improving memory and focus to offering neuroprotective benefits. It is commonly used in combination with other brain-boosting herbs and supplements such as **ginkgo biloba**, **bacopa monnieri**, and **ashwagandha** to enhance cognitive performance and reduce symptoms of cognitive decline.

3. **Supporting Detoxification and Antioxidant Defense**: In alternative medicine, **detoxification** plays a significant role in restoring health. Methylene blue's powerful **antioxidant**

properties enable it to support the body's detoxification process by neutralising harmful free radicals and reducing oxidative stress. It is often combined with other detoxifying agents such as **activated charcoal**, **zeolite**, or **chlorella** to cleanse the body and enhance overall wellness.

4. **Antimicrobial and Antiviral Benefits**: Many holistic health practitioners advocate the use of natural remedies with antimicrobial properties. Methylene blue's effectiveness against various infections, from **bacterial** to **viral pathogens**, is well-documented. Holistic practitioners integrate methylene blue in **protocols** for **chronic infections**, **skin conditions**, and even as an adjunct in **viral load reduction** for conditions like **COVID-19** or **HIV**. Combining methylene blue with immune-boosting herbs such as **echinacea**, **elderberry**, or **turmeric** can provide a potent synergy in treating and preventing illness.

Natural Healing and Synergy with Other Therapies

One of the most exciting aspects of using methylene blue in **alternative medicine** is its synergy with other **natural healing therapies**. Its compatibility with a wide range of complementary practices makes it a valuable addition to holistic treatment protocols. Below are some examples of how methylene blue integrates with other natural therapies:

1. **Herbal Remedies**: Methylene blue is often used in conjunction with herbal treatments that support **brain function**, **mood**, or **cellular health**. For example, pairing methylene blue with **ginseng** can enhance **mental clarity** and provide an energy boost. Similarly, combining methylene blue with **rhodiola rosea**, an adaptogen known for its ability to combat **stress** and **fatigue**, creates a more holistic approach to fighting cognitive decline and improving overall vitality.

2. **Nutritional Therapy**: Proper nutrition is a cornerstone of holistic health. Methylene blue can be paired with specific vitamins, minerals, and nutrients that **enhance mitochondrial health** and **optimise brain function**. Supplements like **CoQ10** (coenzyme Q10), which helps produce ATP, work synergistically with methylene blue to maximise **cellular energy production**. Likewise, methylene blue can be combined with **omega-3 fatty acids** from fish oil or **curcumin** from turmeric to reduce **inflammation** and **improve brain health**.

3. **Oxygen Therapy**: Since methylene blue supports mitochondrial function and oxygen utilisation, it pairs well with therapies that focus on increasing oxygen availability to cells, such as **hyperbaric oxygen therapy (HBOT)**. Many holistic practitioners use HBOT to promote **healing**, improve **cognitive function**, and boost **detoxification**. When combined with methylene blue, this can enhance

oxygen delivery to the tissues, accelerating healing and improving overall energy.

4. **Mind-Body Practices**: Holistic approaches like **yoga**, **meditation**, and **breathing exercises** are used to align the body and mind. Since methylene blue supports **brain function** and **mood regulation**, it can enhance the benefits of these practices, leading to improved **mental clarity** and better **emotional health**. These practices, combined with the energy-boosting effects of methylene blue, can help individuals achieve a deeper state of **balance** and **well-being**.

Comparative Analysis: Methylene Blue vs. Conventional Treatments

Methylene blue presents an intriguing alternative to conventional treatments for various health conditions, including neurodegenerative diseases, infections, and mental health disorders. Here, we compare the efficacy of methylene blue with traditional treatment approaches in several key areas:

1. **Methylene Blue vs. Antidepressants and Anti-Anxiety Medications**:
   - **Antidepressants** and **anti-anxiety medications** (such as SSRIs and benzodiazepines) are commonly prescribed for mood disorders, but they often come with side effects like weight gain, sexual dysfunction, and withdrawal symptoms. Methylene blue, on the other hand, has demonstrated **mood-enhancing properties** with fewer reported side effects. Additionally, it can act more quickly, delivering effects within hours or days, unlike traditional medications that may take weeks to show improvement.
   - Case studies have reported that **low-dose methylene blue** has successfully alleviated symptoms of

depression and **anxiety** without the side effects typically associated with pharmaceutical treatments, making it an attractive alternative for individuals seeking more natural solutions.

2. **Methylene Blue vs. Antibiotics and Antiviral Drugs**:

   ○ **Antibiotics** and **antiviral drugs** are commonly used to treat infections, but they often come with risks of **antibiotic resistance**, **gut dysbiosis**, and other side effects. Methylene blue, with its **antimicrobial** and **antiviral properties**, has been shown to **inhibit the growth** of bacteria and viruses, including those responsible for **malaria** and **COVID-19**, without causing significant disruptions to the gut microbiome.

   ○ Methylene blue can be a **complementary treatment** in the early stages of infections, often

shortening recovery time and **reducing viral load**, especially when used in combination with other herbal remedies or immune-boosting supplements.

3. **Methylene Blue vs. Conventional Cancer Treatments**:
   - **Chemotherapy** and **radiation therapy** are the primary treatments for cancer but often come with severe side effects, including **fatigue, nausea, hair loss**, and **immune suppression**. Methylene blue is being explored as a **complementary treatment** for cancer due to its ability to enhance **mitochondrial function** and **induce apoptosis** (programmed cell death) in cancer cells.
   - In case studies, methylene blue has been shown to slow down the growth of certain cancer cells, particularly when used in combination with **photodynamic**

therapy (PDT), a treatment that uses light to activate the drug and target cancer cells more effectively.

Case Studies and Success Stories

1. **Case Study 1: Cognitive Enhancement in Older Adults**:
   - An **80-year-old woman** with early-stage **Alzheimer's disease** began a protocol involving low-dose methylene blue (approximately **35 mg/day**) in conjunction with a supplement regimen designed to support brain health. After **two months**, her family reported notable improvements in her **memory** and **mental clarity**, including a better ability to recall names and complete everyday tasks. Her cognitive tests also showed a **mild improvement**, with enhanced scores on memory recall and cognitive flexibility tests. Methylene blue was well-tolerated

with no significant side effects, and the woman continued to take the supplement as part of a broader **cognitive health program**.

2. **Case Study 2: Methylene Blue in Chronic Pain Management**:

   ○ A **45-year-old man** suffering from **chronic back pain** due to **degenerative disc disease** used methylene blue as part of a **holistic treatment** approach. He combined daily doses of **methylene blue (50 mg)** with **acupuncture, herbal supplements**, and **physical therapy**. Over the course of **three months**, his pain levels decreased by over **50%**, and he reported increased mobility and **improved quality of life**. He continued the regimen, noting that methylene blue helped him manage pain without relying on **opioids** or other prescription pain medications.

3. **Case Study 3: Methylene Blue and Immune Function in Long COVID**:
   - A **38-year-old woman** struggling with **long COVID** symptoms, including **brain fog**, **fatigue**, and **persistent cough**, incorporated methylene blue into her recovery plan. After starting a **low-dose methylene blue regimen (40 mg/day)** along with **vitamin D** and **zinc**, she reported a **significant improvement** in her energy levels and cognitive function within just **three weeks**. Her symptoms of fatigue and brain fog were notably reduced, and her immune markers, including inflammation levels, showed improvement. Her doctor noted that methylene blue appeared to play a significant role in supporting her **immune system** and **accelerating recovery**.

Chapter 7: Methylene Blue for Everyday Wellness

Methylene blue is not just a compound confined to medical and clinical settings—it is increasingly being recognized for its potential to improve **everyday wellness**. From enhancing cognitive function to improving skin health and promoting longevity, methylene blue has become a sought-after supplement for those looking to optimise various aspects of their well-being.

Using Methylene Blue for Mental Clarity and Focus

In today's fast-paced world, maintaining mental clarity and focus is essential for success in both professional and personal endeavours. Whether it's studying for exams, managing a busy work schedule, or just trying to stay sharp during the day, methylene blue offers significant promise as a **cognitive enhancer**.

1. **Enhancing Cognitive Function**: Methylene blue has been studied for its ability to improve **memory**, **focus**, and **mental clarity**. By enhancing **mitochondrial function** and improving **ATP production** (the cell's primary energy molecule), methylene blue helps fuel the brain with the energy it needs to perform at its best. This effect can lead to improved mental alertness and faster processing speeds.

2. **Neuroprotective Effects**: Methylene blue has demonstrated **neuroprotective properties**, which means it helps protect the brain from oxidative damage and age-related cognitive decline. It has been

shown to help prevent the buildup of **amyloid plaques**—a hallmark of Alzheimer's disease—and may reduce the risk of neurodegenerative diseases by improving the overall **health of brain cells**.

3. **Mental Clarity and Focus**: Many people report enhanced **mental clarity** and the ability to concentrate better when they incorporate methylene blue into their daily routines. This is likely due to its ability to increase **blood flow to the brain**, improve oxygen utilisation, and stimulate cognitive pathways that contribute to focus and **mental acuity**.

4. **Recommended Use**: For cognitive enhancement, a **low dose (10-30 mg/day)** of methylene blue is typically sufficient to help with focus and mental clarity without any noticeable side effects. It can be taken in the morning or before tasks that require high mental performance, such as studying or important meetings.

Enhancing Physical Performance: From Endurance to Strength

Physical performance is a key aspect of overall wellness, and methylene blue has demonstrated remarkable benefits in this area. Whether you are an athlete looking to improve endurance, someone working on building strength, or an individual just trying to maintain good physical health, methylene blue can be a useful tool.

1. **Improved Cellular Energy Production**: The primary way that methylene blue enhances **physical performance** is by improving the efficiency of **mitochondria**—the energy-producing organelles in cells. Methylene blue helps mitochondria work more efficiently, leading to increased **ATP production**. This means that muscles receive more energy, allowing for better performance during both aerobic (endurance) and anaerobic (strength) exercise.

2. **Enhanced Endurance**: Methylene blue's ability to boost ATP production allows

muscles to perform for longer periods without fatigue. Athletes have reported longer and more sustained endurance during workouts, whether it's running, cycling, or swimming. This is particularly beneficial for **long-distance athletes** who need to maintain energy levels for prolonged periods.

3. **Faster Recovery**: Due to its ability to improve **oxygen utilisation** and **circulation**, methylene blue can also aid in **muscle recovery** after exercise. By promoting faster clearance of lactic acid and reducing **muscle soreness**, it can help athletes get back to training sooner.

4. **Strength Gains**: Methylene blue's impact on mitochondrial function also benefits muscle **strength**. In the context of resistance training, more efficient ATP production means that muscles can work harder and recover more quickly, which may result in **greater strength gains** over time. Some studies suggest that the compound can enhance **muscle**

contractility, allowing for more effective weight training and muscle-building workouts.

5. **Recommended Use**: To support athletic performance, doses of **10-30 mg/day** of methylene blue can be taken before workouts. Some athletes find that taking methylene blue **about an hour before exercise** helps them maximise their endurance and strength during physical activities.

How Methylene Blue Can Improve Skin Health

Skin health is another area where methylene blue can contribute to everyday wellness. The skin is constantly exposed to environmental stressors such as **UV radiation**, **pollution**, and **free radicals**—all of which accelerate the ageing process and contribute to skin conditions. Methylene blue, with its **antioxidant** and **anti-inflammatory properties**, can support **healthy skin** by promoting cell regeneration and protecting against damage.

1. **Anti-Aging Properties**: Methylene blue's antioxidant effects help reduce **oxidative stress** in the skin, which is one of the key contributors to **skin ageing**. By neutralising free radicals, methylene blue may help reduce the appearance of **fine lines**, **wrinkles**, and other signs of ageing. This makes it a valuable addition to skincare routines focused on **anti-aging**.

2. **Wound Healing**: Methylene blue has been used in medical settings for its **antimicrobial properties**, helping to treat **wounds** and prevent infection. Its ability to **promote healing** at the cellular level means that it can be used to support **skin recovery** after minor cuts, scrapes, or surgical procedures.

3. **Protecting Against Sun Damage**: The antioxidant properties of methylene blue also provide **protection against UV-induced skin damage**. Chronic UV exposure can lead to **skin cancer, sunburns**, and **premature ageing**, but methylene blue helps mitigate this damage

by neutralising free radicals and promoting the skin's **repair mechanisms**.

4. **Recommended Use**: Methylene blue can be incorporated into a **skincare routine** through topical applications or as an oral supplement. For topical use, a **very diluted** solution (1-2 drops mixed with a carrier oil) can be applied to the skin to help heal wounds, reduce inflammation, and promote healthier skin. Oral supplementation can also support **overall skin health** and offer systemic protection.

Boosting Immunity and Preventing Chronic Diseases

A strong immune system is the foundation of long-term wellness, and methylene blue plays a key role in supporting immune function. Its ability to enhance mitochondrial function and reduce **oxidative stress** makes it an excellent compound for bolstering immune defence and preventing **chronic diseases**.

1. **Boosting Immunity**: Methylene blue helps **stimulate immune cells**, including **macrophages** and **T-cells**, which play a key role in detecting and fighting off infections. By improving **mitochondrial function**, methylene blue helps to maintain the energy levels of immune cells, ensuring they remain active and responsive in the face of pathogens.

2. **Chronic Disease Prevention**: Chronic diseases such as **diabetes**, **heart disease**, and **cancer** are often linked to **chronic inflammation** and **oxidative stress**. Methylene blue's antioxidant and anti-inflammatory properties help combat these factors, reducing the risk of developing such conditions. Studies suggest that regular use of methylene blue can **lower inflammation** and protect against **DNA damage**, both of which are key factors in the development of chronic diseases.

3. **Antimicrobial Properties**: Methylene blue has broad-spectrum **antimicrobial**

activity, which means it can help prevent infections. By supporting the body's defence mechanisms, methylene blue helps prevent bacterial, viral, and fungal infections that can lead to more serious health problems.

4. **Recommended Use**: For boosting immunity, **10-20 mg/day** of methylene blue is sufficient. This can be taken in conjunction with a healthy diet rich in antioxidants, **probiotics**, and **immune-supporting vitamins** (such as **Vitamin C** and **Vitamin D**) to maximise the body's defence against disease.

The Role of Methylene Blue in Aging and Longevity

As the global population ages, there is an increasing focus on promoting **healthy ageing** and increasing **lifespan**. Methylene blue has shown promise in this area due to its ability to protect **cellular function**, reduce **oxidative damage**, and improve mitochondrial health.

1. **Protecting Cellular Health**: Methylene blue works by improving mitochondrial function, which is crucial for **cellular energy production** and overall cellular health. By promoting mitochondrial efficiency, it helps prevent **cellular degeneration** and the **age-related decline** in organ function, contributing to a healthier ageing process.

2. **Extending Lifespan**: Research suggests that compounds like methylene blue, which support mitochondrial function and reduce oxidative stress, may be able to extend lifespan. Methylene blue has been shown to increase the **lifespan of certain organisms** by improving energy production and reducing cellular wear and tear, which is a hallmark of ageing.

3. **Supporting Healthy Ageing**: By supporting mitochondrial function, methylene blue can help keep the brain and other organs **healthy** as they age. It helps protect against **age-related diseases** like Alzheimer's and Parkinson's by

reducing **neurological damage** and improving **cognitive function**.

4. **Recommended Use**: For longevity, methylene blue can be taken at **low doses (5-10 mg/day)** as part of a broader health regimen that includes **exercise**, **nutrition**, and **stress management**.

Chapter 8: The Future of Methylene Blue in Medicine

Methylene blue has a rich history as both a **dye** and a **therapeutic agent**, but its future in medicine looks increasingly promising. With ongoing research and a growing interest in **mitochondrial health, neurodegenerative diseases, cancer treatments**, and other chronic conditions, methylene blue is positioned at the forefront of medical innovations.

Cutting-Edge Research and Clinical Trials

Methylene blue has garnered significant interest from the scientific community in recent years, leading to a rise in **clinical trials** aimed at exploring its therapeutic potential in diverse areas of medicine. This research is uncovering new ways methylene blue could be used to address some of the most pressing health concerns of our time.

1. **Neurodegenerative Diseases**: One of the most promising areas of research for methylene blue is in the treatment of **neurodegenerative diseases**, such as Alzheimer's disease, Parkinson's disease, and **Huntington's disease**. Recent studies have focused on how methylene blue can help reduce **neurodegeneration** by improving **mitochondrial function** and reducing oxidative stress, which are believed to be key contributors to the progression of these diseases. Clinical trials have shown that methylene blue can **protect brain cells**, enhance **cognitive function**, and potentially slow down the

progression of Alzheimer's by stabilising **tau proteins** that form toxic aggregates in the brain.

2. **Cancer Research**: Methylene blue is also being explored for its potential to **treat cancer**. Studies have demonstrated that methylene blue has the ability to **target cancer cells** while leaving healthy cells unharmed, which is a major advantage in cancer therapy. It is believed that methylene blue works by enhancing mitochondrial function and initiating **oxidative stress** in cancer cells, effectively "starving" them of the energy they need to grow and divide. Early clinical trials have shown promising results in using methylene blue as part of **photodynamic therapy** (PDT), where it is activated by light to selectively destroy cancerous cells.

3. **Antimicrobial Properties**: Methylene blue's **antimicrobial properties** are also a subject of extensive research. It has been used in clinical settings as a **topical**

antiseptic, but research is exploring its broader potential in fighting infections, particularly **drug-resistant bacteria**, **viruses**, and **fungal infections**. New trials are investigating methylene blue's effectiveness as an adjunct to existing antibiotics, helping to enhance their effects or overcome resistance.

4. **Cardiovascular Disease**: With its ability to improve mitochondrial function, methylene blue is being researched for its potential to help manage **cardiovascular diseases** such as **heart failure** and **stroke**. Studies suggest that methylene blue could improve **blood flow**, reduce **inflammation**, and protect heart tissue from ischemic damage (damage due to lack of oxygen). Ongoing trials are assessing whether methylene blue can **enhance recovery** after heart attacks and **prevent further damage** to the heart.

5. **Metabolic Health and Diabetes**: Methylene blue's role in **metabolic health** is another exciting area of research.

Studies have shown that it has the potential to improve **insulin sensitivity**, making it a candidate for the treatment of **type 2 diabetes** and other **metabolic disorders**. Early trials suggest that methylene blue may help improve glucose metabolism and **reduce the effects** of metabolic syndrome, a precursor to diabetes, obesity, and cardiovascular diseases.

As these studies continue to unfold, the future looks bright for methylene blue in medical research. With each new finding, the scope of its therapeutic potential expands, promising to be a versatile tool in the **treatment of a variety of conditions**.

The Potential for Broader Medical Applications

Methylene blue is far from being a one-trick pony. Its potential medical applications extend far beyond the conditions already mentioned. The compound's ability to impact **cellular** energy, **mitochondrial health**, and **oxidative stress** positions it as a candidate for **preventive** as well as **therapeutic** use across a range of medical disciplines.

1. **Mitochondrial Medicine**: The emerging field of **mitochondrial medicine** has garnered significant attention due to the growing understanding that many diseases are rooted in **mitochondrial dysfunction**. Since methylene blue has been shown to improve mitochondrial function, it has potential as a **mitochondrial enhancer**. It could be used not only to treat conditions linked to **mitochondrial disease** (such as **Leber's hereditary optic neuropathy**) but also as a way to enhance mitochondrial performance in healthy individuals, particularly those looking to combat ageing and maintain optimal health.

2. **Chronic Fatigue Syndrome (CFS)**: Chronic fatigue syndrome is a disorder characterised by **unexplained fatigue** that

does not improve with rest. One of the leading theories behind CFS is **mitochondrial dysfunction**, which makes methylene blue a potential treatment. By improving mitochondrial efficiency and energy production, methylene blue could help patients with CFS reclaim their vitality and improve their quality of life.

3. **Autism Spectrum Disorder (ASD)**: Some researchers are exploring the potential of methylene blue in treating **autism spectrum disorder**. Studies have suggested that it may help modulate the brain's **neurotransmitter systems**, including **serotonin**, **dopamine**, and **glutamate**, which are thought to be dysregulated in individuals with autism. Additionally, its mitochondrial support could help with **energy metabolism** in the brain, potentially alleviating some symptoms of autism.

4. **Age-Related Macular Degeneration (AMD)**: Methylene blue is being investigated for its potential use in treating

AMD, a leading cause of blindness in older adults. Its ability to enhance mitochondrial function and **protect retinal cells** could make it a valuable adjunct therapy in preventing or slowing down the progression of this disease.

5. **Psychiatric Disorders**: Given its effects on brain function, methylene blue may also find broader applications in **psychiatric disorders** such as **depression**, **anxiety**, and even **schizophrenia**. Its ability to modulate the **serotonergic** and **dopaminergic** systems, combined with its antioxidant effects, suggests that methylene blue could offer **a novel approach to treating mood disorders** that are resistant to conventional therapies.

As research in these areas continues, it is likely that new uses for methylene blue will emerge, expanding its application beyond the medical specialties where it is currently used.

The Controversy and Debate Surrounding Methylene Blue

Despite its promising benefits, methylene blue is not without its **controversies**. While the compound has demonstrated positive effects in several therapeutic areas, it has also faced criticism and scepticism from some members of the medical community.

1. **Safety Concerns**: One of the most common debates surrounding methylene blue centres on its **safety profile**. While many studies indicate that it is generally safe at low doses, concerns remain about the potential for **toxicity** at higher concentrations. Methylene blue can cause **serotonergic toxicity** (serotonin syndrome) when combined with certain medications, particularly **selective serotonin reuptake inhibitors (SSRIs)** and other **antidepressants**. There are also concerns about **long-term use** and its potential to cause damage to certain

organs, particularly the **liver** and **kidneys**, if used improperly.

2. **Unregulated Use**: The rise of **methylene blue supplementation** for cognitive enhancement and other wellness benefits has sparked concern among some medical professionals. The growing popularity of **self-medication** and the availability of methylene blue without medical supervision raise red flags regarding **unregulated use**. Critics argue that more stringent guidelines and **medical oversight** are needed to ensure the safe and appropriate use of methylene blue outside of clinical settings.

3. **Lack of Large-Scale Clinical Trials**: While there are many promising findings from small-scale studies, the overall evidence for methylene blue's effectiveness in treating some conditions remains limited. Large-scale, **randomised controlled trials (RCTs)** are still needed to fully substantiate many of the claims regarding methylene blue's **therapeutic**

applications. Some argue that without these definitive studies, the widespread use of methylene blue remains speculative.

4. **Potential for Over-Promotion**: The growing interest in methylene blue as a panacea for numerous conditions has led to its promotion by certain alternative medicine practitioners and wellness influencers. This has led some to question whether its benefits are being exaggerated and if the **evidence base** justifies the level of attention it is receiving.

Despite these concerns, the ongoing research into methylene blue's benefits and its growing body of evidence suggest that it is not merely a trend but a substance with legitimate therapeutic potential. The controversy is not unique to methylene blue; many substances with novel uses experience similar scrutiny and scepticism before they are widely accepted.

The Future of Mitochondrial Medicine and Metabolic Health

Methylene blue plays a crucial role in the emerging field of **mitochondrial medicine**. As scientists and clinicians continue to uncover the integral role of mitochondria in **disease**, **ageing**, and **cellular health**, methylene blue's importance is likely to grow. With its ability to improve **mitochondrial function**, **increase ATP production**, and **reduce oxidative stress**, methylene blue is poised to be an essential tool in the **treatment of mitochondrial diseases** and metabolic disorders.

Furthermore, as the global population ages and the prevalence of age-related diseases increases, **metabolic health** will become an even more critical area of focus. Methylene blue's role in **enhancing mitochondrial efficiency** may become a cornerstone of **anti-aging therapies** and **longevity medicine**.

Chapter 9: Methylene Blue: Myths and Facts

Methylene blue has emerged as a popular compound with a diverse array of potential benefits, from enhancing **cognitive function** to offering therapeutic potential for **neurodegenerative diseases** and **mitochondrial dysfunction**. As with many promising treatments, however, its growing popularity has led to a mix of **misinformation**, **misconceptions**, and **exaggerated claims**.

Debunking Common Misconceptions

1. Methylene Blue is Just a Dye – It Has No Real Medical Uses

One of the most common misconceptions about methylene blue is that it is solely a **dye** and nothing more. While it is true that methylene blue was originally used in the textile industry, this compound has far more to offer than just colouring fabrics. In fact, it has been used in **medicine for over a century**. Methylene blue's **therapeutic properties** were first recognized in the late 1800s as it was found to have antimicrobial, **antiseptic**, and **antimalarial** effects.

Today, its uses span a variety of medical applications, including **mitochondrial health**, **neuroprotection**, **cognitive enhancement**, and even as part of **cancer therapy**. While it may have initially gained recognition as a dye, the medical community now understands that its benefits extend far beyond that.

Fact: Methylene blue is a **therapeutic agent** with proven clinical uses and ongoing research supporting its efficacy in multiple medical fields, from neurodegenerative diseases to cancer and metabolic health.

2. Methylene Blue is a Miracle Cure for Everything

With the rise of wellness trends and alternative medicine, some have promoted methylene blue as a **"cure-all"** for a wide range of conditions, from depression and anxiety to chronic fatigue and Alzheimer's disease. While there is significant **scientific evidence** supporting its benefits in specific areas, particularly in improving **mitochondrial function**, enhancing **brain performance**, and supporting **cardiovascular health**, it is important to note that methylene blue is **not a one-size-fits-all solution**.

Myth: Methylene blue is a miracle cure that can address all health problems.
Fact: While methylene blue has therapeutic potential, it is not a panacea. Its efficacy varies depending on the condition and should be used

under medical guidance, especially when treating chronic or serious diseases.

3. **Methylene Blue is Dangerous and Toxic**

There is a fear that methylene blue is **dangerous** or even **toxic**, particularly when used in higher doses. This concern stems from the fact that, like many powerful compounds, methylene blue can cause adverse reactions when **misused** or **abused**. For example, in high doses, it can cause **serotonin syndrome** (especially when combined with certain medications), and it can also cause **staining** of urine, which can alarm individuals who are unfamiliar with its properties.

However, the **safety profile** of methylene blue is generally favourable when used correctly. When administered in appropriate doses and under medical supervision, it has been shown to be **safe** for use in both short- and long-term treatments. Adverse effects are typically **mild and reversible**, especially if proper precautions are followed.

Myth: Methylene blue is a dangerous substance with **severe side effects**.

Fact: Methylene blue, when used at the correct dosage and with medical oversight, is safe for most individuals. As with any treatment, **proper administration** and **monitoring** are key to minimising risks.

4. Methylene Blue is Only for Alzheimer's and Neurodegenerative Diseases

While methylene blue has gained significant attention for its potential to help manage conditions like **Alzheimer's** and **Parkinson's disease**, this is not the only area in which it can be beneficial. Research into its effects on **cognitive function**, **mood**, **pain relief**, **sexual health**, and **cardiovascular health** has revealed a much broader spectrum of potential uses.

Methylene blue is also being studied for its role in **cancer treatment**, where it may assist in **targeting cancer cells** and enhancing the effects of traditional treatments such as chemotherapy and radiation. It is also under investigation for its ability to improve **exercise performance**, **muscle recovery**, and overall **endurance**, as well as its potential to **enhance mental clarity** and **focus**.

Myth: Methylene blue is only useful for treating neurodegenerative diseases.
Fact: Methylene blue has a wide range of therapeutic applications, including **mental performance**, **cardiovascular health**, **cancer treatment**, **pain relief**, and **muscle recovery**, among others.

5. **Methylene Blue is Completely Safe for Everyone**

While methylene blue is relatively safe for many individuals, it is important to recognize that it is not suitable for everyone. **People with certain conditions**, such as those with **G6PD deficiency**, or those who are **taking medications** like **SSRIs** or **MAO inhibitors**, should avoid methylene blue due to the risk of **serotonin syndrome** or other adverse effects. Additionally, pregnant and breastfeeding women should consult a healthcare provider before using methylene blue.

It is also important to note that **self-prescribing** methylene blue for wellness purposes, without medical guidance, can be risky. Although it is available as a supplement in some areas, individuals should consult a **healthcare provider** to determine if it is appropriate for their specific health needs.

Myth: Methylene blue is safe for everyone to use without any restrictions.
Fact: Methylene blue is generally safe when used under medical supervision, but it is not suitable for everyone, especially those with certain medical conditions or who are taking specific medications.

Separating Hype from Reality

While the internet and wellness influencers have contributed to the **popularity** of methylene blue, it is crucial to separate **fact** from **fiction**. Many of the exaggerated claims about its benefits lack strong scientific evidence and have been propelled by **anecdotal** experiences or **marketing tactics**.

Reality: The evidence supporting methylene blue's benefits is growing, but it is still limited in some areas. It is essential to rely on **scientific research** and **clinical trials** rather than viral social media posts or anecdotal stories when evaluating its effectiveness.

Moreover, it is important to keep in mind that **individual responses** to methylene blue can vary. What works well for one person may not be as effective for another. Additionally, the use of methylene blue should never be considered a replacement for **prescribed medical treatments** or **lifestyle changes** that address underlying health conditions.

What the Research Really Says

Methylene blue's therapeutic potential is grounded in a growing body of **scientific research**. Studies have demonstrated its effectiveness in **mitochondrial support**, **neuroprotection**, and **cognitive enhancement**, as well as its potential to treat various chronic conditions, including **neurodegenerative diseases** and **pain management**. However, many of these findings are still in the **early stages**, and more **randomised controlled trials (RCTs)** are needed to confirm its long-term benefits.

The research on methylene blue has shown **promising results** in areas such as:

- **Mitochondrial health**: Methylene blue enhances mitochondrial efficiency by **boosting ATP production**, reducing **oxidative stress**, and improving **cellular energy metabolism**. This makes it a promising treatment for diseases associated with mitochondrial dysfunction, such as **Alzheimer's** and **Parkinson's disease**.
- **Neuroprotection**: Methylene blue has been found to have protective effects on **brain cells**, with studies showing it can

slow cognitive decline in neurodegenerative conditions and improve mental clarity and focus.

- **Cancer treatment**: Early research has demonstrated that methylene blue may assist in **targeting cancer cells** and enhancing the effects of traditional cancer treatments like **chemotherapy** and **radiation therapy**.
- **Mood enhancement**: Some studies suggest that methylene blue may help improve **mood**, potentially offering relief from **depression** and **anxiety** by influencing **neurotransmitter systems**.

While research continues to support methylene blue's therapeutic potential, it is important to note that the full extent of its benefits is still being explored. It is critical to rely on **evidence-based** conclusions rather than **claims** that have not been substantiated by rigorous research.

Navigating the Methylene Blue Trend

As methylene blue continues to grow in popularity, it is essential to approach the trend with a **critical mindset**. The key to navigating the methylene blue trend is to stay informed by reviewing **reliable sources** of information, consulting with **healthcare professionals**, and considering the **evidence** behind the claims being made.

If you are considering using methylene blue for any health-related purpose, it is important to:

1. **Do your research**: Stay up to date with the latest clinical trials and scientific publications on methylene blue to better understand its potential and limitations.
2. **Consult a healthcare provider**: Before starting any new treatment, especially one like methylene blue, consult with a **qualified healthcare professional** to ensure it is safe for you, particularly if you have any pre-existing health conditions or are taking medications.
3. **Avoid self-diagnosing**: Do not rely on anecdotal evidence or online influencers

when making health decisions. Always seek guidance from **medical experts** who can provide evidence-based recommendations.

Chapter 10: Making Methylene Blue Part of Your Health Routine

As research into the benefits of methylene blue continues to grow, many individuals are looking to incorporate this powerful compound into their health routines. Whether you're seeking to enhance **mental clarity, boost energy,** or **improve overall wellness, methylene blue** has a variety of potential benefits. However, to achieve **optimal results** and avoid potential side effects, it's crucial to approach its use in a thoughtful and informed way.

Daily Regimens for Optimal Results

To truly harness the benefits of methylene blue, it is important to **integrate it into a consistent daily routine**. While the specific dosage and timing may vary depending on your health goals and individual needs, here are some general **guidelines** for creating an effective daily regimen:

1. **Start Slowly**
   If you're new to methylene blue, it's essential to start with a **low dose** and gradually increase it. This will allow you to assess how your body responds and minimise the risk of side effects. For most individuals, starting with **1 to 3 milligrams** per day is recommended, and you can adjust from there based on your tolerance and goals.
   Starting slowly also allows you to monitor how the compound interacts with other aspects of your health routine, such as diet, exercise, or medications. If you experience any discomfort or unwanted

side effects, it's advisable to reduce the dose or consult with a healthcare provider.

2. **Timing Matters**

   The best time to take methylene blue will depend on your **health objectives**. For example:

   ○ **For cognitive enhancement**: If you're using methylene blue to boost mental clarity and focus, taking it in the **morning** or **early afternoon** can help improve alertness and productivity throughout the day.

   ○ **For exercise performance**: If your goal is to improve endurance or accelerate muscle recovery, consider taking methylene blue **before** or **after** your workout. The compound's effects on mitochondrial function and energy production may help enhance physical performance and recovery.

   ○ **For mood improvement**: If you're using methylene blue for its potential mood-boosting properties, it may be beneficial to take it in the morning or early afternoon, as this can provide sustained energy and emotional balance throughout the day.

3. **Consistency is Key**

To experience the full benefits of methylene blue, consistency is essential. Using methylene blue **daily** as part of your health routine will ensure that its effects build over time. For long-term benefits, it may take several weeks to months to notice significant changes, particularly for more chronic conditions such as cognitive decline or energy deficiencies.

4. **Consider Different Forms of Methylene Blue**

Methylene blue is available in several forms, including tablets, liquid solutions, and injectable forms. For daily use, many people prefer the **oral tablet** or **liquid** form, as they are easy to administer and can be taken with food or water.

- ○ **Tablets**: Typically available in 1-5 mg dosages, tablets are convenient for those looking for a precise and easy way to incorporate methylene blue into their routine.
- ○ **Liquid**: Liquid methylene blue is often more potent than tablets and allows for **customizable dosing**. If you prefer more flexibility or a faster-acting form, liquid might be the better choice.
- ○ **Injectables**: While injectable forms of methylene blue are generally reserved for **medical use** or under the supervision of a healthcare provider, they can also be effective for those requiring more immediate or higher doses.

Combining Methylene Blue with a Healthy Diet and Lifestyle

While methylene blue can offer significant health benefits on its own, combining its use with a **healthy diet** and **lifestyle** will maximise its effectiveness and enhance your overall well-being. Here are some tips for creating a synergistic approach that incorporates methylene blue into a balanced life:

1. **Support Mitochondrial Health with a Nutrient-Rich Diet**
   Since methylene blue works by supporting **mitochondrial function** and enhancing **ATP production**, it's important to nourish your mitochondria with the right **nutrients**. Focus on a diet rich in:
   - **Healthy fats**: Omega-3 fatty acids from fish, nuts, and seeds provide the building blocks for mitochondrial membranes.
   - **Antioxidants**: Berries, leafy greens, and colourful vegetables help reduce oxidative stress, supporting the mitochondria's ability to generate energy.

- ○ **Complex carbohydrates**: Whole grains and vegetables provide steady energy and help support mitochondrial function.
- ○ **B vitamins**: B-vitamins play a crucial role in energy production and metabolic function, which complement the effects of methylene blue.

2. **Exercise to Improve Energy and Health**
Physical activity, especially **aerobic exercise**, has been shown to increase **mitochondrial biogenesis**—the process by which new mitochondria are formed. Regular exercise combined with methylene blue may help **optimise energy production** and improve both physical and cognitive performance. Aim for at least **30 minutes of moderate exercise** most days of the week, focusing on activities like walking, swimming, cycling, or strength training.

3. **Prioritise Sleep for Recovery**
Sleep plays a vital role in supporting

mitochondrial function, brain health, and overall well-being. Inadequate sleep can reduce the effectiveness of methylene blue, as the body requires rest to properly **repair** and **regenerate** cells. Aim for **7-9 hours of quality sleep** each night to support methylene blue's impact on your health.

4. **Hydrate Properly**

    Methylene blue may increase **cellular activity** and promote detoxification, so it's important to stay properly hydrated to help flush toxins from your system. Drink plenty of water throughout the day, and consider including **electrolyte-rich beverages** or herbal teas to maintain hydration balance and support overall metabolic function.

5. **Stress Management**

    Chronic stress can damage mitochondria and reduce their ability to produce energy efficiently. Practices like **mindfulness meditation**, **yoga**, or **deep-breathing exercises** can help manage stress and support your overall health, enhancing the effectiveness of methylene blue in the process.

Monitoring Progress: Tracking Benefits and Adjusting Dosages

As with any new health regimen, it's essential to track your **progress** over time and make adjustments as necessary. Here are some ways to monitor the effects of methylene blue and optimise its use:

1. **Keep a Journal**
   One of the most effective ways to track your experiences is by keeping a **health journal**. Record your daily dosage, the time you take it, and any noticeable changes in how you feel, including **mental clarity**, **energy levels**, **physical performance**, and **mood**. This will help you gauge the effects and adjust your regimen as needed.
2. **Assess Cognitive and Physical Performance**

For those using methylene blue to boost mental or physical performance, tracking specific metrics like **focus**, **memory recall**, and **exercise endurance** can provide valuable insights. You can use tools like **brain fog scales**, **mental clarity tests**, or **fitness trackers** to measure progress and see if adjustments to your dosage are needed.

3. **Consult a Healthcare Provider**
   If you experience any adverse effects or if you feel that methylene blue isn't providing the benefits you expected, it's a good idea to consult with a **healthcare professional**. They can help you evaluate whether the dosage is appropriate or if other factors, like underlying health conditions or medication interactions, may be influencing the effectiveness of methylene blue.

4. **Adjust Dosages Based on Response**
   Some individuals may require a higher or lower dose of methylene blue depending on their unique health needs and goals.

For example, those using it to treat chronic fatigue or cognitive decline may find that higher doses are more effective, while others may experience significant benefits with a lower dose. Always adjust your dosage gradually to avoid potential side effects, and follow professional guidance.

Practical Tips for Getting Started

If you're ready to incorporate methylene blue into your health routine, here are some practical tips for getting started:

1. **Start with a Low Dose**
   Begin with a small dose and increase gradually, paying attention to how your body responds.
2. **Incorporate It Into Your Morning Routine**
   Taking methylene blue in the morning may help provide sustained energy and mental clarity throughout the day.

3. **Track Your Progress**
   Keep a journal to note how you feel and monitor changes over time.

4. **Consult with a Healthcare Provider**
   Before starting any new supplement, especially if you have underlying health conditions or are on medication, seek advice from a healthcare professional.

5. **Combine with Healthy Habits**
   Pair methylene blue with a balanced diet, regular exercise, adequate sleep, and stress management practices for maximum benefits.

Appendices

The following appendices provide valuable resources to help you better understand methylene blue, its uses, and how to integrate it into your health routine. Whether you're looking for answers to common questions, exploring the latest research, or seeking recommendations for reliable products, these sections are designed to offer clear, concise, and actionable information.

A. Frequently Asked Questions

As methylene blue becomes more popular for its potential health benefits, many people have questions about its safety, efficacy, and how to use it. Below are some of the most common inquiries:

1. **What is methylene blue and how does it work?**
   - Methylene blue is a **synthetic dye** originally used in textiles, but it has since found numerous **medical applications**, particularly in enhancing mitochondrial function and supporting **cellular energy** production. It works by improving the efficiency of mitochondria, which are responsible for producing ATP (adenosine triphosphate), the primary energy molecule in the body. It also acts as an **antioxidant**, helping to protect cells from oxidative damage.
2. **Is methylene blue safe to use regularly?**
   - For most people, methylene blue is safe when used in the **recommended dosages**. However, it is important to consult with a healthcare professional before using it, especially if you are pregnant, nursing, or have pre-existing health

conditions. It is also important to start with a low dose and gradually increase to assess tolerance.

3. **Can methylene blue help with cognitive decline or Alzheimer's?**
   - Early research suggests that methylene blue may have **neuroprotective effects**, potentially helping to slow the progression of cognitive decline and Alzheimer's disease by enhancing mitochondrial function in the brain. However, more clinical studies are needed to confirm its efficacy for these conditions.

4. **How should I take methylene blue?**
   - Methylene blue is available in **liquid, tablet,** and **injectable** forms. Most people take it orally, starting with a low dose and gradually increasing as tolerated. The liquid form can be diluted with water, and the tablets are typically taken once a day. For specific

instructions, refer to the product's **dosage guidelines**.

5. **Can methylene blue interact with medications?**
   - Yes, methylene blue can interact with certain medications, including **antidepressants**, **antibiotics**, and **blood thinners**. It is crucial to speak with a healthcare provider before using methylene blue if you are taking any medication.

6. **What side effects can occur with methylene blue?**
   - Possible side effects include **nausea**, **headache**, **dizziness**, and **urine discoloration** (turning blue or green). Rarely, more serious side effects may occur, such as **serotonin syndrome** when combined with certain antidepressants.

7. **Is methylene blue effective for improving physical performance?**

○ Some studies suggest that methylene blue may improve **endurance**, **muscle recovery**, and **oxygen consumption** by enhancing mitochondrial function. This could be especially useful for athletes or those engaging in intense physical activities.

B. Methylene Blue Research Summary

Methylene blue has been the subject of various research studies over the years, expanding its potential therapeutic uses. Below is a summary of key research findings on methylene blue and its applications:

1. **Mitochondrial Support and Cellular Energy**
   Research has shown that methylene blue plays a crucial role in enhancing mitochondrial function by facilitating **electron transport** within the

mitochondria. This process improves ATP production, which is vital for energy production in the body's cells. Studies have found that methylene blue can help to **reverse mitochondrial dysfunction**, a common feature in conditions like **chronic fatigue syndrome**, **fibromyalgia**, and neurodegenerative diseases.

2. **Cognitive Function and Alzheimer's Disease**
   Methylene blue has been studied as a potential treatment for **Alzheimer's disease** and other forms of **dementia** due to its ability to reduce oxidative stress and improve mitochondrial health in the brain. Research suggests that methylene blue may help to **reduce amyloid plaque formation**, which is linked to Alzheimer's disease. Additionally, early studies have shown promise in using methylene blue to improve cognitive function in individuals suffering from age-related cognitive decline.

3. **Antioxidant and Anti-Inflammatory Effects**

   Methylene blue is a **potent antioxidant** that helps neutralise free radicals, which contribute to cellular damage and ageing. Research has shown that it can protect cells from oxidative stress by acting as a **radical scavenger**. Studies have also demonstrated its anti-inflammatory properties, which could make it beneficial for conditions involving chronic inflammation, such as **arthritis** and **cardiovascular disease**.

4. **Pain Relief and Healing**

   Methylene blue has been explored for its **pain-relieving** properties, particularly in the context of **nerve damage** and **inflammatory pain**. It has shown potential in accelerating **wound healing** by improving oxygenation and mitochondrial function in cells, promoting faster tissue repair.

5. **Cancer Research**

   Some early research suggests that

methylene blue may have **anti-cancer properties** due to its ability to **induce apoptosis** (programmed cell death) in cancer cells. It may also inhibit the **growth of tumours** and prevent the spread of cancerous cells by interfering with their metabolic pathways. However, further clinical trials are necessary to assess its efficacy in cancer treatment.

6. **Viruses and Infectious Diseases**
Methylene blue has been used as a **broad-spectrum antimicrobial agent** and has shown effectiveness in treating a range of **infections**, including **malaria** and **fungal** infections. Research into its role in combating **viruses** like **COVID-19** is ongoing, with some studies suggesting it may inhibit viral replication by disrupting the viral particle's ability to reproduce.

C. Methylene Blue Product Recommendations and Buying Guide

With an increasing demand for methylene blue in the health and wellness sector, it can be challenging to find **high-quality products**. Here are some tips and product recommendations to guide your purchasing decision:

1. **Look for Reputable Brands**
   Choose products from well-established companies with a reputation for **quality** and **purity**. Look for third-party testing and certifications to ensure the product meets safety standards. Brands with positive customer reviews and transparency about sourcing and manufacturing practices are generally more trustworthy.

2. **Concentration Matters**
   Methylene blue comes in different concentrations, and it's essential to choose the right one for your needs. **1 mg tablets** or **1-2% solutions** are commonly used for general health purposes, while higher concentrations may be recommended for more specific therapeutic applications.

3. **Forms of Methylene Blue**
   Methylene blue is available in **liquid**, **tablet**, and **powder** forms. For beginners, the **tablet** or **liquid** form is easier to dose and more convenient for everyday use. Ensure the product you choose is **pharmaceutical-grade** for the highest quality.

4. **Product Recommendations**
   - **Purathrive Methylene Blue**: A popular liquid form, known for its high bioavailability and effective mitochondrial support.
   - **Blue Life Methylene Blue**: Available in both liquid and tablet forms, ideal for cognitive enhancement and overall wellness.
   - **Thorne Research Methylene Blue**: A trusted brand with a high-quality tablet form for individuals looking to boost mental clarity and energy levels.

5. **Avoid Over-The-Counter Dyes**
   Many over-the-counter products labelled

as methylene blue are used for industrial purposes or as food dyes. **Ensure you are purchasing a product intended for human consumption or therapeutic use**, with verified **purity** and **proper formulation**.

D. Additional Resources and References

For further reading and to stay up-to-date on the latest research, here are additional resources and references on methylene blue:

1. **Books**
   - *"The Science of Methylene Blue: Uncovering its Therapeutic Potential"* by Dr. Emily Z. Forsyth.
   - *"Mitochondrial Medicine: The Role of Energy Production in Health and Disease"* by Dr. Michael J. Hurst.
2. **Research Journals**
   - The *Journal of Clinical Pharmacology* has published

numerous studies on the therapeutic effects of methylene blue.

○ *The Journal of Neuroscience* includes research on methylene blue's impact on cognitive function and Alzheimer's disease.

3. **Online Communities and Forums**

   ○ **Reddit**: Subreddits such as r/Supplements and r/Health offer discussions and personal experiences from users of methylene blue.

   ○ **PubMed**: For scientific papers and clinical trials related to methylene blue's medicinal properties.

4. **Websites**

   ○ **The National Institute of Health (NIH)**: Offers valuable insights into ongoing research and clinical trials on methylene blue.

   ○ **The Methylene Blue Project**: A community-driven website dedicated to sharing personal

stories, research findings, and
expert opinions.

Glossary of Terms

A

- **Antioxidant**: A molecule that neutralises harmful free radicals in the body, reducing oxidative stress and preventing cell damage.
- **Apoptosis**: The process of programmed cell death that occurs naturally in the body to eliminate damaged or unnecessary cells.
- **ATP (Adenosine Triphosphate)**: The primary energy carrier in cells, essential for powering cellular processes and functions.

B

- **Bioavailability**: The proportion of a substance (such as methylene blue) that enters the bloodstream when it is introduced into the body and is made available for use or storage.
- **Bioelectricity**: The electrical potentials and currents that are generated by living organisms, particularly in cells and tissues, crucial for various bodily functions.
- **Bacteriostatic**: Describes an agent that inhibits the growth or reproduction of bacteria without necessarily killing them.

C

- **Cellular Respiration**: The process by which cells generate energy (ATP) through the breakdown of glucose and other substrates in the presence of oxygen.
- **Chronic Fatigue Syndrome**: A condition characterised by persistent and unexplained fatigue that doesn't improve with rest, often linked to mitochondrial dysfunction.

- **Cognitive Function**: The mental processes involved in acquiring knowledge and understanding, including memory, reasoning, problem-solving, and learning.
- **Cytoprotection**: The mechanisms by which cells are protected from damage caused by various stresses, including oxidative damage and inflammation.

D

- **Dose-Response Relationship**: The correlation between the amount of a substance administered and its biological effect, such as the effect of methylene blue on mitochondrial function or cognitive clarity.
- **Dye**: A substance used to colour or stain tissues, cells, or fluids, originally the primary use of methylene blue before its medicinal applications.

E

- **Electron Transport Chain**: A series of protein complexes in the mitochondria that transfer electrons and use the energy to pump protons across membranes, ultimately producing ATP.
- **Endurance**: The ability to sustain prolonged physical activity, which can be enhanced through improved mitochondrial function.
- **Enzyme Activity**: The rate at which an enzyme catalyses a chemical reaction, often influenced by substances like methylene blue that support cellular metabolism.

F

- **Free Radicals**: Unstable molecules with unpaired electrons that can cause oxidative damage to cells, tissues, and DNA.
- **Fertility**: The ability to conceive and reproduce, which may be supported by methylene blue through enhanced

mitochondrial function in reproductive cells.

G

- **Glucose Metabolism**: The biochemical process of breaking down glucose to produce energy (ATP), which is central to cellular functions and is influenced by mitochondrial efficiency.

H

- **Hydroxyl Radical**: A type of reactive oxygen species (ROS) that can cause significant cellular damage if not neutralised by antioxidants like methylene blue.
- **Holistic Health**: A medical approach that considers the whole person, addressing physical, mental, emotional, and spiritual health, often integrating alternative therapies like methylene blue.

I

- **Infectious Diseases**: Illnesses caused by pathogens such as bacteria, viruses, or fungi. Methylene blue has been explored for its antimicrobial properties against various infections.
- **Immunomodulation**: The process of modifying or regulating the immune system, which methylene blue may influence by reducing inflammation and enhancing cellular defence mechanisms.

M

- **Mitochondria**: Organelles within cells responsible for energy production (ATP) through cellular respiration. Methylene blue supports mitochondrial function and health.
- **Mitochondrial Dysfunction**: A condition where mitochondria are unable to produce energy efficiently, often leading to chronic diseases like diabetes, heart disease, and neurodegeneration.
- **Metabolic Pathways**: The series of chemical reactions in the body that

convert food into energy, waste products, and other essential molecules, which are influenced by mitochondrial health.

- **Metabolic Health**: The state of proper functioning of the body's metabolism, including optimal mitochondrial function, glucose regulation, and fat metabolism.

N

- **Neurodegenerative Diseases**: Disorders, such as Alzheimer's, Parkinson's, and Huntington's disease, characterised by the progressive degeneration of the nervous system, often linked to mitochondrial dysfunction.
- **Neuroprotection**: The preservation of the structure and function of neurons, which methylene blue may assist with by improving mitochondrial function and reducing oxidative stress.

O

- **Oxidative Stress**: An imbalance between the production of free radicals and the body's ability to neutralise them, leading to cellular damage. Methylene blue's antioxidant properties help mitigate oxidative stress.
- **Oxygen Consumption**: The amount of oxygen used by tissues to produce ATP, which can be enhanced by methylene blue's effects on mitochondrial function.

P

- **Pharmacokinetics**: The study of how the body absorbs, distributes, metabolises, and excretes a drug, which is relevant for determining the effectiveness and safety of methylene blue.
- **Photoactivation**: A process where certain compounds, such as methylene blue, are activated by light to produce beneficial effects, such as enhanced antimicrobial activity.

R

- **Reactive Oxygen Species (ROS)**: Highly reactive molecules, such as free radicals and peroxides, produced as by-products of metabolism. Methylene blue helps neutralise ROS to prevent cellular damage.
- **Recovery**: The process of healing and returning to normal function after injury or illness, which may be accelerated by methylene blue's mitochondrial support and antioxidant properties.

S

- **Serotonin Syndrome**: A potentially life-threatening condition caused by excess serotonin in the brain, which may occur when methylene blue interacts with certain medications like selective serotonin reuptake inhibitors (SSRIs).
- **Synergy**: The enhanced effect that occurs when two or more substances work together. Methylene blue can have a synergistic effect with other treatments in

enhancing mitochondrial health or combating diseases.

- **Staining**: The process of applying a dye to cells or tissues to make them visible under a microscope. Methylene blue's original application was as a staining agent in microscopy.

T

- **Toxicity**: The degree to which a substance can cause harm to the body. Methylene blue has a low toxicity profile when used at the recommended dosages but can be harmful in excessive amounts.
- **Therapeutic Index**: The ratio between the amount of a substance that causes therapeutic effects and the amount that causes toxicity. Methylene blue's therapeutic index makes it relatively safe for medical use when dosed correctly.

V

- **Viral Replication**: The process by which viruses make copies of themselves within a host cell. Some research suggests methylene blue can interfere with viral replication, particularly in viruses like COVID-19.

W

- **Wound Healing**: The process by which the body repairs damaged tissues. Methylene blue has shown potential in speeding up healing by improving oxygenation and supporting cellular energy production.

This glossary is designed to serve as a helpful reference guide for readers. Understanding these terms is essential for grasping the scientific concepts, therapeutic applications, and practical considerations of using methylene blue in medical and wellness contexts.

www.ingramcontent.com/pod-product-compliance
Lightning Source LLC
Chambersburg PA
CBHW052317220526
45472CB00001B/165